Urinalysis and Body Fluids for
CLS & MLT

Mary Michelle Shodja, PhD, MS, CLS (ASCP)

Order this book online at www.trafford.com
or email orders@trafford.com

Most Trafford titles are also available at major online book retailers.

Print information available on the last page.

ISBN: 978-1-4907-8937-8 (e)
ISBN: 978-1-4907-8938-5 (sc)

Our mission is to efficiently provide the world's finest, most comprehensive book publishing
service, enabling every author to experience success. To find out how to publish your book,
your way, and have it available worldwide, visit us online at www.trafford.com

Trafford rev. 06/20/2018

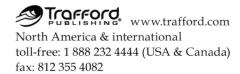

www.trafford.com
North America & international
toll-free: 1 888 232 4444 (USA & Canada)
fax: 812 355 4082

To my mother, for her sacrifices, this is for you.

To my best friend of almost 30 years, Anna Liza Hamilton, thank you for being there through the good times and the bad, I look forward to many more years of friendship. To my sisters, Mae, Chingbee and Lee thank you for your continued love and support. Lastly, with deep gratitude to Christine Sy, Chona Aros and Helena Pangan, thank you for being a part of my life.

"That which does not kill me makes me stronger"
Friedrich Nietzsche

To laboratory students and fellow laboratorians, never forget what you learned and never stop learning new things.
The Author

Preface

This manual is the seventh of a series of 20 manuals that the author was commissioned to write for the Medical Laboratory Technology (MLT) training program in Diamond Bar, California that was granted approval as a training facility in 2009 by the State Department of Health and Human Services. In writing these manuals, the author strived to adhere to the strict guidelines of the State of California's requirements for the MLT program.

The author revised these manuals to serve 3 purpose: as the primary textbooks for the 6-month MLT training program, as reviewers for Clinical Laboratory Scientists (CLSs) preparing for the CLS Licensure or Certification, and as a continuing education materials for CLSs and MLTs as a requirement for license renewal.

The author wrote these manuals in an outline form for easy reading and understanding and free from the constraint of a formal textbook. The author's intention is to speak to the reader from the actual clinical laboratory bench than from the classroom.

The Urinalysis and Body Fluids for CLS and MLT only discussed the most common urinary diseases and body fluids encountered in the clinical laboratory and are not intended as a replacement to the actual textbooks currently being employed in the CLS program.

Also by Mary Michelle Shodja, PhD, MS, CLS (ASCP)

Bacteriology for CLS & MLT
Hematology for CLS & MLT
Parasitology for CLS & MLT
Mycology for CLS & MLT
Coagulation for CLS & MLT
Virology for CLS & MLT
Routine Chemistry for CLS & MLT
Special Chemistry for CLS & MLT
Toxicology for CLS & MLT
Serology – Immunoassays for CLS & MLT
Serology – ELISA Assays for CLS & MLT
Serology & Syphilis for CLS & MLT
Immunology for CLS & MLT
Blood Bank for CLS & MLT
Phlebotomy for CLS & MLT
Specimen Processing for CLS & MLT
Laboratory Safety for CLS & MLT
Total Quality Management I – Quality Assurance
Total Quality Management II – Quality Control

Contents

List of Pictures

SECTION I: Introduction to Urinalysis

The urinalysis test is used as a screening and/or diagnostic tool because it can help detect substances or cellular material in the urine associated with different metabolic or kidney disorders. Together with the complete blood count (CBC) test, urinalysis is one of the most commonly ordered laboratory test in the hospital. Certain substances like glucose and protein may be detected first before the appearance of any signs or symptoms. Urinalysis is used mainly to detect Urinary Tract Infection (UTI) and other disorders of the urinary tract in patients with acute or chronic conditions.

Indications for Urinalysis test includes:

a. Abdominal pain
b. Back pain
c. Frequent or painful urination
d. Blood in the urine

Urinalysis is composed of the chemical portion and the microscopic portion.

Definitions:
- Polyuria – urine volume > 2,000 ml/24 hours
- Olyguria – urine volume of < 500 ml/24 hours
- Anuria – no urine production

SECTION II: The IRIS® Automated Urine Chemistry Analyzer

Because urinalysis is one of the most commonly ordered laboratory test, the 10-analyte tests embedded in a strip called a "dipstick" that composed the chemical portion of the urinalysis is usually performed using an automated reader or analyzer. Although the dipstick could be read manually it is not only cumbersome, the manual reading my sometimes be subjective and could be time consuming. Larger hospitals also employ an automated microscopic analyzer to standardize the process, as well as keep a permanent documentation of the readings.

Although there are a number of automated urinalysis analyzers, the most popular among them is the IRIS® Automated Urinalysis System and will be discussed here in detail. It is an in-vitro diagnostic system composed of the AX-4280 chemistry module, the iQ200 microscopy module, a computer and a monitor. The system is used to automate the complete routine urinalysis test.

The IRIS® AX-4280 instrument is several steps up from the more common and simpler urinalysis analyzers that mainly uses spectrophotometer to measure the color change on the pads and calculates the results. The IRIS® AX-4280:

- Determines the color by comparison to 4 light waves of different colors
- Determines clarity of the specimen by passing a light beam through the sample and measuring the scattered light
- Determines the specific gravity (mass of a specific volume) by measuring the refraction angles of the light
- Performs the chemistry panel consists of 9 elements:
1. Glucose
2. Protein
3. Bilirubin
4. Urobilinogen
5. pH
6. blood
7. ketones
8. nitrite
9. leukocytes

- Principle – measures the chemical constituents using the Aution® test sticks which are read by a dual wavelength reflectance system. The Aution® test strip contains 9 pads impregnated with chemicals specific for the determination of a particular constituent. A correction pad is included on the strip to compensate for the natural color of urine and its effect on the color reactions of the reactive pads. Test strips are dispensed from the test strip feeder and placed on the test strip tray. The sample probe aspirates an aliquot of urine and dispenses it onto the test pads, color changes and the intensity of reflected light from the reactive pads is measured spectrophotometrically. These measurements are used to calculate clinically meaningful results.

- Quality Control (QC) – should be run daily.

SECTION III: The IRIS®
Automated Microscopic Analyzer

The iQ200 instrument

- Performs the microscopic portion of the urinalysis and provides qualitative or quantitative count of formed elements such as cells, casts, crystals, and organisms. The system photographs particles as they are passed in front of the camera. The images are classified, counted and stored for review by the users.
- The workstation consists of a computer that is interfaced with the AX-4280 and iQ200. The chemistry and microscopic results could be viewed and the microscopic results could be edited in the same frame.
- Principle – urine specimens are mixed and a portion is aspirated and is sandwiched between enveloping layers of a suspended fluid called "lamina" which is positioned exactly within the depth and field of the view of the objective lens of a microscope that is coupled to a video camera.
- QC – is required daily.

Workstation

- Specimen results are reviewed and edited as needed. Images are classified as:
  WBC – White Blood Cells
  RBC – Red Blood Cells
  Bacteria
  Epithelial cells
  Calcium oxalate crystals
  Amorphous crystals

THE OPERATOR CAN FURTHER CLASSIFY:
UNCX – unclassified crystals
UNCC – unclassified casts
NSE – Non-squamous epithelial cells
BYST – yeast

 MARY MICHELLE SHODJA, PHD, MS, CLS (ASCP)

SECTION IV: Macroscopic Appearance

Urine Specimen Collection

- Vaginal or penile area should be cleansed with the sterile disposable moist towellete
- First morning specimen is the best specimen
- Midstream collection is the best method
- Sterile urines include:

Suprapubic collection – collection by needle aspiration
From the bladder
From the kidney
In and out catheter

- Storage – refrigerated up to 24 hours
- Testing – at room temperature

The macroscopic examination of urines may yield important information regarding the patient's condition.

CLEARNESS OR CLOUDINESS

- Clear = fresh
- Turbid – below are possible causes:
  Alkaline urine (pH>7.0) has phosphates and carbonates
  Acid urine (pH<7.0) has urates and uric acid
  Bacteria
  WBCs
  RBCs
  Sperm
- Milky
  Chyluria – presence of lymphocytes in the fluid
  Pyuria – increased number of leukocytes in the urine
- Oily
  Lipiduria
  Contaminants

COLOR OF URINE

a. Colorless – very dilute
b. Yellow – urochrome (end product of hemoglobin breakdown), uroerythrin (pinkish or reddish pigment seen in many pathological urines)
c. Yellow-brown-green – bilirubin, biliverdin (foam)
d. Red – porphyrin, blood, hemoglobin, myoglobin
e. Brown-black – melanin, homogentisic acid, methemoglobin
f. Blue-green – Pseudomonas, indicant (precursor of indigo dye)

ODOR OF URINE

a. Aromatic – fresh
b. Ammonia – old specimen, bacterial contamination
c. Fruity – diabetes mellitus
d. Mousy – phenylketonuria

SECTION V: Urine Chemistry

There are 10 analytes that commonly comprised the urine chemistry test. This section discussed all 10 tests and its significance.

<u>pH</u>

- Significance includes:
    a. >8.5 – indicates bacterial infection
    b. <6.5 acid urine caused by high protein diet, diet with acidic fruits, acidosis, hypokalemia, acidic drugs
    c. >6.5 and <8.5 – alkaline urine caused by diet rich in vegetables, citrus, dairy products, alkalosis, impaired tubular function, bacterial infection, alkaline drugs
    d. pH affects stone formation, cast preservation and efficiency of certain antibiotics
    e. Commonly used reference range: 4.5-8.0
    f. Principle: use of a color indicator is sensitive to H^+ concentration (methyl red and bromcresol blue)- Result of yellowish indicates acidic, bluish indicates basic

<u>SPECIFIC GRAVITY (SG)</u>

- Significance includes:
    a. Evaluation of diluting or concentrating ability of kidney
    b. Measures the total solute concentration
    c. Proportional to number of weight of dissolved compounds
- ↓SG
  Excessive water intake
  Diabetes insipidus
  Tubular damage
- ↑SG
  Dehydration
  Increased antidiuretic hormone production
  Glucosuria
  Heart failure
  Liver failure

Renal disease
- Formula: Weight of 1 ml of urine/weight of 1 ml of water
- Commonly used reference range: 1.003-1.030
- Principle: Refractrometer (gold standard) or Dipstick (Color change)

Refractrometer device:
Refractive Index (RI) = velocity of light in air/velocity of light in solution

Dipstick:
pK_a of pretreated polyelectrolytes changes in relation to ionic concentration, color change from deep blue-green to green or yellow-green

FALSE NEGATIVES occur in pH>6.5

Urinometer:
Rarely used
Uses weighted device placed in liquid
Must subtract 0.001 for every 3 degrees below 22^0C and must add 0.001 for every 3 degrees above 22^0C
Must calibrate against distilled water each day of use (value=1.000)

SPECIFIC GRAVITY AND OSMOLALITY

- Both are related to the quantity of solutes in the urine
- If the patient is to be evaluated for renal concentration ability, urine osmolality should be used since it is a more accurate measurement of quantity of total solutes present
- Osmolality is not as commonly requested as specific gravity
- Osmolality commoly used reference range: 50-1200 mOsm/kg water

NITRITE

Significance:
- Detects presence of growth of most bacteria (some bacteria that are nitrate negative are not detected)
- Reference range: Negative
- Principle: Dietary nitrate is converted to nitrite by bacteria with the enzyme bacterial reductase (mostly gram negative organisms)

Reagent strip has P-arsanilic acid + nitrite →diazonium salt
Diazonium salt + benzoquinoline →pink azodye

Pink color = positive
False negative – infection with bacteria that does not convert nitrite to nitrate (Enterococcus faecalis, Streptococcus, Staphylococcus saprophyticus), absence of dietary nitrate, ascorbic acid >25mg/dL
False positive – none except red colored materials

WBC's

Significance:
- Detects presence of white blood cells in urine by measuring the presence of leukocyte esterase. Leukocyte esterase is present in the primary granules of neutrophils
- Indicates urinary tract infection (UTI) or other inflammatory conditions causing elevated WBCs in urine
- Reference range: Negative
- Principle: Reagent strip method
  Leukocyte esterase + indoxyl carbonic acid →ester indoxyl = O_2 indigo + diazonium salt→purple chromogen
- False negatives – contamination with genital tract WBCs, formalin

PROTEIN

Significance:
- Excess of protein in urine
- Commonly used reference ranges: 40-150 mg/24 hours, 5-10 mg/100 ml, dipstick methods are designed to read "within normal limit" at approximately 20 mg/100 ml or below
- As much as 30 grams of protein filters into the glomerular filtrate each day. Thus it would be a great metabolic drain on the body if protein were not returned to the body fluids
- Normally, it is the smaller molecular weight (primarily albumin, <30,000 daltons) that flow into the glomerular filtrate. Larger proteins stay in the efferent arterial and are not filtered into the filtrate
- Because protein molecule is much too large to be transported by the usual transport processes, protein is absorbed through the brush border of the proximal tubular epithelium by pinocytosis, by simply attaching itself to

the membrane and this portion of the membrane then invaginates to the interior of the cell

- Once inside the cell, the protein is probably digested into its constituent amino acids, which are then actively absorbed through the base of the cell into the peritubular fluids
- High molecular weight (HMW) protein loss (>60,000 daltons) = glomerular damage
- Low molecular weight (LMW) protein loss (<30,000 daltons) = tubular damage
- Types of proteinuria:
    a. Functional – associated with fever, exposure to cold, dehydration, emotional stress or severe and unaccustomed exercise. Proteinuria is transient and apparently benign, although may persist up to 3 days after severe exercise
    b. Orthostatic – proteinuria on certain individuals when standing and disappears when lying down, no clinical significance
    c. Pre-renal – proteinuria due to primarily to a disease other than kidney disease, e.g. Multiple Myeloma (MM)
    d. True proteinuria – proteinuria in which some of the protein elements of the blood are discharged in the urine
    e. Tamm-Horsefall protein – a glycoprotein normally excreted by the kidneys into the urine. About half of the normal urinary proteins are Tamm-Horsefall protein, the rest is albumin. Tamm-horsefall protein holds the cellular elements in casts together
- Diseases and their relation to the amount of renal proteinuria:
    a. Heavy >4g/day – nephrotic syndrome
    b. Moderate 1-4 g/day – glomerular disease
    c. Mild <1g/day – chronic renal disease
- Reference range: Negative
- Principle:
    a. Reagent Strip: Simple colorimetric test that employs the pH indicator. Bromcresol blue is yellow at pH 3.0 but with protein present, the color becomes green-blue

Although not as sensitive as precipitation test, this test has the advantage of avoiding false positive reactions with organic iodides as used in renal pyelography and false positives with tolbutamide or other drugs

b. Precipitation method – with heat and acetic acid, with nitric acid and with sulfosalicylic acid (SSA), or trichloroacetic acid (TCA). In most clinical laboratories, a positive protein dipstick test is confirmed with precipitation method, the most common is the SSA.

False positive – pseudo-proteinemia – all of the acid precipitation tests will give false positive results when organic iodine x-ray media are present. Urinary excretion may persist for 3 days after administration of the dye.

Using Trichloroacetic Acid (TCA) can be more sensitive to small amounts of protein and can be measured by turbidometry or can be dissolved in nitric acid and reacted with ammonium hydroxide to produce a yellow color, which is measured photometrically.

TCA is a protein precipitant that causes gamma globulin to be precipitated with a greater turbidity than with albumin.

Sulfosalicylic Acid (SSA) precipitates protein in urine with a turbidometry that is approximately proportional to the concentration of protein in a solution and may be measured with a photometer.

With SSA, turbidity produced with albumin is 2-3x that produced with a globulin. Polypeptide proteins and Bence-Jones proteins are also precipitated.

Bence- Jones protein
  ◦ Represents the light chain of the abnormal immunoglobulins found in multiple myeloma
  ◦ This protein precipitates between the temperatures 40 and 60^{0}C and re-dissolves again near 100^{0}C if the concentration of Bence-Jones is too great
  ◦ The best method to measure Bence-jones proteins is by protein electrophoresis, immunoelectrophoresis (IEP) and immunofixation (IF). A homogenous band in the globulin region will be seen on paper or cellulose acetate

Mucin
- Mucoid and nucleoproteins present in normal urine only in traces. Inflammation or irritation of urogenital tract mucous membrane cause increased amounts. Can be mistaken for albumin.
- Mucin test – white cloud forms when urine diluted with water and acidified with acetic acid.

RBCs

- Hematuria – discharge of blood in the urine, finding of intact RBCs in the urinary sediment either grossly visible as a reddish color on the urine or RBCs microscopically or in a cast
- Substances giving the urine a reddish color includes the following:
    a. Hemoglobin
    b. Myoglobin
    c. Porphyrin
    d. Methemoglobin
    e. Phenolphthalein
    f. Rhubarb (group of plant of the genus Rheum, Senna a large genus of >250 species of flowering plants), Cascara (a plant known for its laxative properties)

Etiology
    a. Traumatic – flank or abdominal injuries, stab wounds, surgery, bladder puncture
    b. Inflammatory – cystitis (UTI-E. coli, TB, Schistosomiasis, mechanical catheterization)
    c. Urethritis
    d. Prostatitis – usually Mycoplasma infection
    e. Pyelitis – (inflammation of renal pelvis) or pyelonephritis (UTI that had reached the nephrons)
    f. Glomerulonephritis – large category of renal diseases characterized by morphologic changes in the glomerular tufts. Causes include: post-streptococcal, post-viral infection, Systemic Lupus Erythmatosus, malignant hypertension, Goodpasteur's Syndrome
    g. Neoplastic – affecting all areas of urinary tract
    h. Vascular
    i. Obstructive – calculi
    j. Congenital – anatomic abnormalities

k. Other:
   Vigorous exercise
   Associated with febrile disease
   Orthostatic hematuria in adolescents
   Contamination by menses
- Diagnosis of hematurias
   a. Gross appearance – clots, gross blood, urine color is red, pink or red-brown
   b. Microscopic – RBCs, RBC casts (usually suggest kidney as the origin), RBCs mixed with WBCs indicate a variety of processes, tumor cells
   c. Precautions – often rbc cells are missed (if it is destroyed, only the hemoglobin will be detected but you can't see the intact RBCs), yeast cells may be mistaken for RBCs
   d. Dipstick tests do not necessarily distinguish between hemoglobin and myoglobin or intact RBCs. Microscopy is therefore important

- Commonly used reference range: negative - 1,000 RBCs/ml every 12 hours
- Principle:

Dipstick – H_2O_2 + tetra methyl benzidine (action of heme) -> oxidized chromogen + H_2O

- False negative – large quantities of ascorbic acid or Vitamin C inhibits the reaction
- Hemoglobinuria – presence of hemoglobin (Hgb) in the urine without necessarily the presence of red cells. Intravascular hemolysis overwhelms haptoglobin resulting in free Hgb in serum which is then excreted in the urine. Conditions that increases RBC destruction includes:
   a. Hemolytic states – all hemolytic anemias (Glucose-6-phosphate dehydrogenase deficiency, hereditary spherocytosis, paroxysmal cold hemoglobinuria, March hemoglobinuria, malaria, sulfa drugs)
   b. Hemoglobin will also appear in the urine if red cells lyse in the specimen
- Myoglobinuria – the muscle molecule is small in size and filters through the glomerulus and appears in the urine. Often, the serum is normal in color and the mechanism of renal damage is unknown. This will react positively in the blood dipstick but no RBC seen microscopically

- Myoglobin – an iron protein compound present in the sarcoplasm of striated skeletal and cardiac fibers, structurally similar to hemoglobin but smaller in size, and function as oxygen transport and storage
- Causes of myoglobinuria:
  a. Crash injury
  b. Excessive muscle strain
  c. Extensive infarction – post-Myocardial infarction (MI)
  d. Polymositis (many muscle inflammation)
  e. Hyperthermia (elevated body temperature)
  f. Convulsions
- Laboratory detection of myoglobin
  a. Spectrophotometric absorption at 581 nm
  b. Myoglobin casts
  c. Precipitation by ammonium sulfate removes myoglobin or treatment with sulfosalicylic acid removes other muscle protein
  d. Electrophoresis
  e. Immunoassay

HEMOSIDERIN

- A storage form of iron, aggregates of ferritin, found in bone marrow and reticuloendothelial (RE) system (liver, spleen, nodes)
- Hemosiderinuria – conditions of chronic intravascular hemolysis (hemolytic anemias). Filtered hemoglobin and methemoglobin is reabsorbed and broken down into glomerular tubule cells. The cells accumulate iron in the form of hemosiderin granules. When these cells are shed into urine, hemosiderinuria ensues. Excessive body iron stores e.g. hemochromatosis, excessive transfusions.
- Detection of Hemosiderinuria:
  a. Unstained are refractile brown intracellular elements
  b. Prussian Blue stains for iron and iron in the urine sediment will appear blue with this stain

BILIRUBIN

Bile pigments in urine
- Through the degeneration of hemoglobin, the major bile pigment, bilirubin is formed.

- Bilirubin is the breakdown product of the heme portion of hemoglobin.
- Only Direct Bilirubin will spill into the urine.
- Reference range: Negative
- Principle:
  Diazo Method: Bilirubin coupled to *p*-nitro-benzene diazonium-p-toluene sulfonate to form a blue or purple color. Will detect 0.05-0.1 mg/100 ml.

  Oxidation Method: formation of biliverdin by oxidation producing a green color and a positive test

  Pyridium – a drug used to help fight urinary tract infections, gives a yellow-orange color to urine and can cause difficulty in reading dipstick color reactions. In this situation, the area surrounding the dipstick pads will also be discolored.

  Urine positive for bilirubin needs confirmation, the confirmation test is called Ictotest®. The test is a direct measurement for the presence of bilirubin in the urine.

UROBILINOGEN

- Urobilinogen is bacterially metabolized direct bilirubin which is recirculated after gut absorption. Porphobilinogen and Urobilinogen are increased in urine in acute porphyrias.
- Reference range: 0.2 (Negative)
- Principle:
  Urobilinogen:

  Urobilinogen + Ehrlich's reagent→colored aldehyde that is soluble in Chloroform

  Porphobilinogen:

  Porphobilinogen + Ehrlich's reagent→colored aldehyde that is Insoluble in chloroform

- Porphyrins in urine

- ◦ Porphyrins – a group of diseases where there is a defect in the manufacture of the heme molecule that can result in some heme precursors spilling into the urine
- ◦ Many of these heme precursors fluoresce under Ultra Violet (UV) light
- ◦ These can be detected by acidifying the urine with glacial acetic acid, extracting it with ethyl acetate and then placing the extract under ultraviolet (UV) light (Wood's Lamp). A lavender to violet color in the ethyl acetate fraction indicates the presence of porphyrins.

CARBOHYDRATES

- Basic Structure of Carbohydrates (CHO) are substance that contain C, H and O
- Most sugars have 6 carbons in them

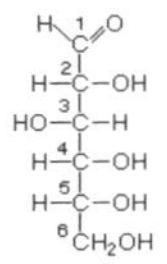

D-Glucose

Picture 1

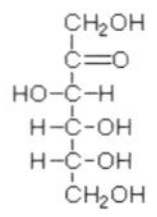

Fructose

Picture 2

- Reducing Sugars or substances that can reduce certain metal ions such Fe^{3+} and Cu^{2+} under the proper conditions, usually alkaline conditions
- It is the aldehyde or ketone group that makes it possible for sugars to be reducing substances
- Disaccharides
  a. Maltose = Glucose + Glucose
  b. Lactose = Glucose + Galactose
  c. Sucrose = Glucose + Fructose
- Diabetes Mellitus
  a. The most common disease involved with carbohydrate metabolism
  b. DM is not related to Diabetes Insipidus (ADH deficiency)
  c. DM is a disease where insufficient insulin is secreted
  d. Insulin forces glucose that is present in the blood into the tissues:
    ↓insulin ↑blood glucose ↑glucose in tissue
    ↑insulin ↓blood glucose ↓glucose in tissue

- Glucose can normally present in urine in small amounts [(<30 mg/dL or "within normal limits") no change in color in the dipstick]
- Glucose passes on into the glomerular filtrate but is then reabsorbed
- A normal fasting glucose is 70-105 mg/dL, when serum glucose reaches 180 mg/dL, then the kidney cannot reabsorbed all the glucose and therefore, glucose "spills" into the urine
- A serum glucose of 180 mg/dL is the renal threshold
- The kidney of diabetics could become more efficient in absorbing glucose and may have a higher renal threshold of up to 240 mg/dL
- Causes of glycosuria (glucose in urine)
    a. DM – most common
    b. Cushing's Syndrome (excess glucocorticoids)
    c. Acromegaly (excess growth hormone)
    d. Hyperthyroidism
    e. Other pancreatic disease resulting in decreased insulin
    f. Excess catecholamines
    g. Renal glycosuria – if there is a defect involving the proximal convoluted tubule (PCT) such that glucose cannot be reabsorbed, then glucose will spill into the urine with normal serum glucose levels. This condition is called Renal Glycosuria, which can result to kidney damage and may have some hereditary association
- Glucose may affect Specific Gravity, Osmolality and Urine Volume results by:
    a. SG and osmolality are both measurements of the amount of solute present in the urine. Glucose will elevate the amount of total solute and will increase SG and osmolality. SG is increased 0.004 for each mg/dL of glucose
    b. The osmolar effect of increased glucose causes the patient to become thirsty
    c. Diabetics therefore excrete large volumes of urine with a higher specific gravity than would be expected
- Reference range: Negative
- Principle: Glucose Oxidation reaction
Glucose + O_2 (through the action of glucose oxidase) →gluconolacetone (H_2O_2 + O_2)→gluconic acid + H_2O_2 + ortho-dianisidine (through the action of peroxidase)→chromogen + H_2O

False negative on large quantities of ascorbic acid (Vitamin C)

False positive on chlorine/hypochlorite contamination and peroxide contamination

- Other methodologies includes Copper Reduction method – false positive in the presence of large quantities of ascorbic acid and large quantities of cephalosporins, chlorine/hypochlorite contamination and false negative on peroxide contamination

Galactosuria
- Some infants are born with inability to metabolize galactose and galactose accumulates and the infant does not thrive and thus treated with lactose-free diet (milk-free). Lactose is a disaccharide made up of glucose and galactose. There is a legal requirement for testing newborns for galactosemia by most states including California.
    a. Lack or deficient in galactose-1-phosphate uridyl transferase (most common), incidence 1:80,000
    b. Lack or deficient galactokinase (less common), incidence is 1:500,000
- Principle:
    a. Galactose level can be measured directly by an RBC enzyme method and by paper chromatography
    b. Galactose may also react positively with Copper reduction methods of measuring sugars (e.g. Benedict's Test)
- Galactose and glucose are the 2 sugars in the urine with the most clinical significance

Fructose
- Lack of enzyme fructokinase, fructose-1-phosphate aldolase
- Incidence is 1:130,000
- Can be measured by paper chromatography and also by resorcinol test
- Resorcinol Test (Selivanoff's Test) – specific for fructose
- Principle:
Fructose + HCl→Hydrozymethylfurfural (action of Resorcinol)→red precipitate

Sucrose
- Sucrose = Fructose + glucose
- A non-reducing sugar because both reducing groups are used in the chemical bond between glucose and fructose

Lactose
- Lack of enzyme lactase, causes diarrhea, abdominal pain, gas
- Lead Acetate Test
  Lactose + Lead acetate in $NH_4OH\rightarrow$Red precipitate
  Note: Glucose causes a yellow precipitate in this test
- Lactose may be present in the urine of pregnant women

Other sugars:
- Other sugars that could be present are pentose (xylulose) due to the lack of xylitol dehydrogenase, 1:2,000 among the Jewish population
- The reference method for identifying non-glucose sugars is Thin Layer Chromatography (TLC)

Benedict's Test (Clinitest)
- Is a non-specific method of measuring all reducing substances in urine including reducing sugars. It is a Copper reduction method.
  $CuSO_4$ (blue) + Reducing Substances $-\rightarrow$ CuOH (yellow)
  CuOH + heat $-\rightarrow$ Cu_2O (red)

  The Clinitest tablet contains copper sulfate, sodium hydroxide, carbonate with a specific test for galactose

Non-sugar Reducing Substances in the urine
  a. Uric acid
  b. Ascorbic acid (Vitamin C – affects several urinalysis chemical tests)
  c. Creatinine
  d. Ketone bodies
  e. Salicylates

If the glucose test on the dipstick is positive, and the reducing sugar is negative, then anyone of the above non-reducing substances may have affected the glucose result.

KETONE
- The body normally uses glucose as its energy source. In situations that the body is deprived of Carbohydrates (CHO), the body will then start breaking down adipose tissue (fat) at a very rapid rate.
- The rapid breakdown of fat causes an accumulation of acetoacetate
- Acetoacetate breaks down to acetone + hydroxybutyrate
- These compounds are acidic which results in metabolic acidosis

- Relative concentration of ketone bodies:
    a. Acetoacetate 20%
    b. Acetone 2%
    c. hydroxybutyrate 78% - major ketone body
- decrease carbohydrate intake or not enough CHO available to the cells may be caused by:

    a. Uncontrolled DM – increase in glucose in the blood but not enough in the tissue because of the lack of insulin to take it there which results to fats breaking down to provide an energy source for the tissue cells
    b. Acute febrile and toxic illnesses, vomiting and diarrheal states, starvation, alcoholic ketoacidosis
- Reference range: Negative

- Principle:
  2 common methods that will both react strongly with acetoacetate, slightly with acetone and no reaction with hydroxybutyrate:
    a. Acetest – Nitroprusside tablet
    b. Ketostix – Nitroprusside on the strip pad
       Nitroprusside is also known as Sodium nitroferricyanide

Normal urine constituents excreted in g/24 hours

Urea	25-30
Uric acid	0.6-0.7
Creatinine	1.0-1.2
Hippuric acid	0.7
Ammonia	0.7
Amino acids	3
Sodium	1-5
Potassium	2-4
Calcium	0.2-0.3
Magnesium	0.1
Chloride	7
Phosphate	1.7-2.5
Sulfate	1.8-2.5

SECTION VI: Microscopic Examination

Microscopic examination of the urine sediment is performed to look for formed cellular elements, casts bacteria, yeasts, parasites and crystals.
- On 10x magnification, check at least 10 fields and look for casts, crystals and squamous epithelial cells
- On 50x magnification, check at least 10 fields and look for RBCs, WBCs, yeasts, bacteria and crystals

CASTS
Picture 3 - Hyaline Cast

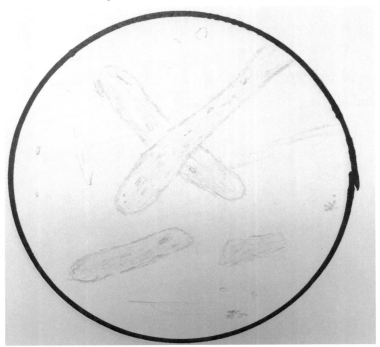

- Tubular secretion of Tamm-Horsefall protein that aggregates into fibrils
- Clinical significance – glomerulonephritis, pyelonephritis, chronic renal disease, congestive heart failure, stress and exercise
- Reference range: 0-2/lpf

Picture 4 - RBC Cast

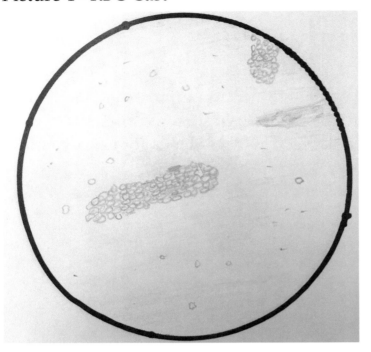

- RBCs enmeshed in or attached to Tamm-Horsefall protein matrix
- Clinical significance – glomerulonephritis, strenuous exercise
- Reference range: 0/lpf

Picture 5 - WBC Cast

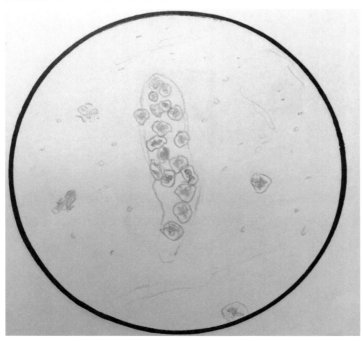

- WBCs enmeshed in or attached to Tamm-Horsefall protein matrix
- Clinical significance – pyelonephritis, acute interstitial nephritis
- Reference range: 0/lpf

Picture 6 - Bacterial Cast

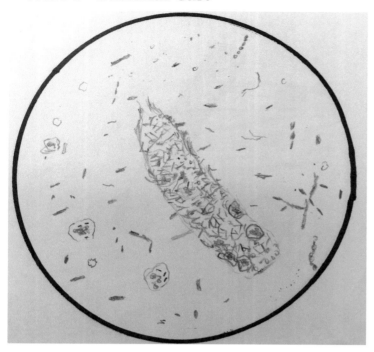

- Bacteria attached to Tamm-Horsefall protein matrix
- Clinical significance – pyelopnephritis
- Reference range: 0/lpf

Picture 7 - Epithelial Cell Cast

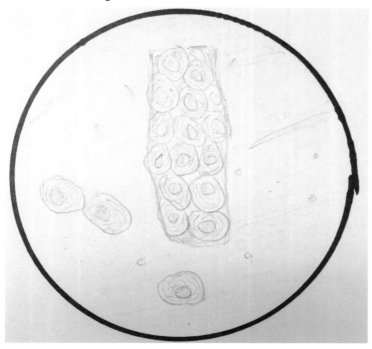

- Tubular cells remaining attached to Tamm-Horsefall protein fibrils
- Clinical significance – renal tubular damage
- Reference range: 0/lpf

Picture 8 - Granular Cast

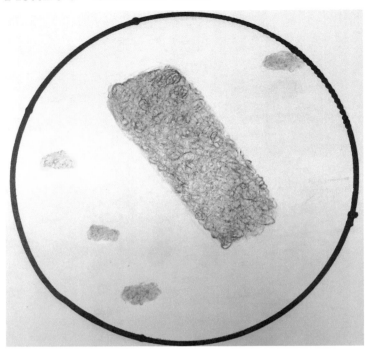

- Disintegration of cellular casts, tubule cell lysosomes, protein aggregates
- Clinical significance – glomerulonephritis, pyelonephritis, stress and exercise
- Reference range: 0-2/lpf

Picture 9 - Waxy Cast

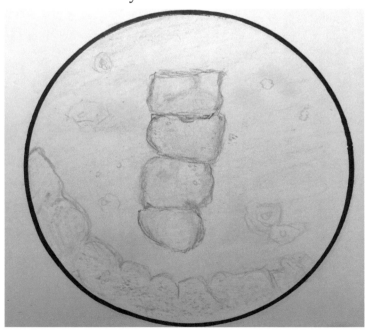

- Hyaline and granular casts
- Clinical significance – stasis of urine flow
- Reference range: 0/lpf

Picture 10 - Fatty cast

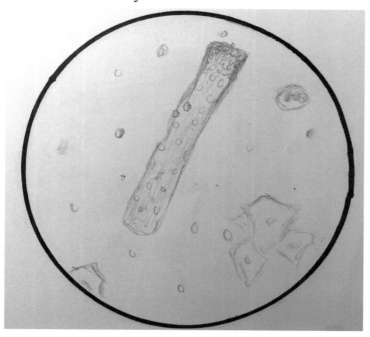

- Urinary lipids, oval fat bodies
- Clinical significance – nephrotic syndrome
- Reference range: 0/lpf

Picture 11 - Broad Cast

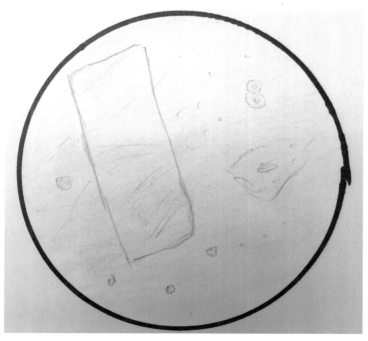

- Formation in collecting ducts or distended distal tubules
- Clinical significance – extreme stasis of flow

CRYSTALS (NORMAL)
Picture 12 - Uric acid

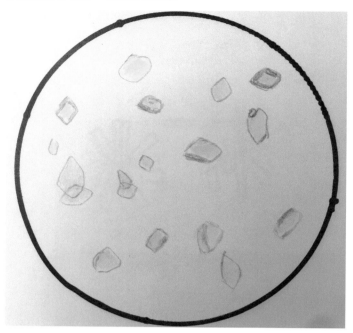

- Acid pH
- Yellow-brown
- Solubility: alkali

Picture 13 - Amorphous crystals

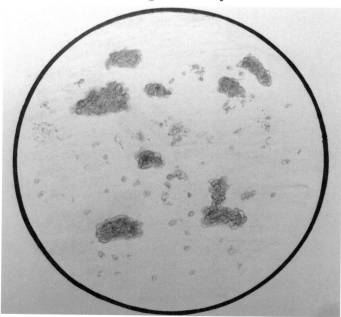

- Acid pH – amorphous urates, alkali and heat soluble
- Brick dust or yellow
- Alkaline pH – amorphous phosphates, dilute acetic acid soluble
- White-colorless

Picture 14 – Calcium oxalate dihydrate

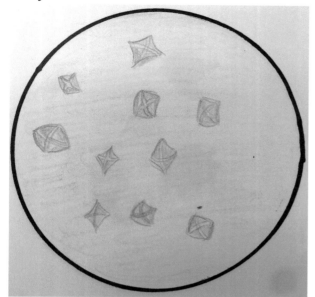

Picture 15 – Calcium oxalate monohydrate

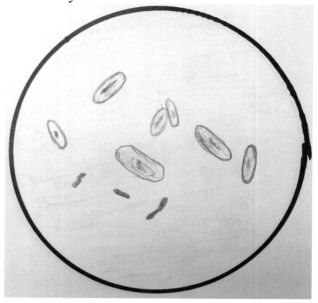

Calcium oxalate dehydrate
- Acid/neutral pH
- Colorless
- Solubility: dilute HCl

Calcium oxalate monohydrate

Picture 16 - Calcium phosphate

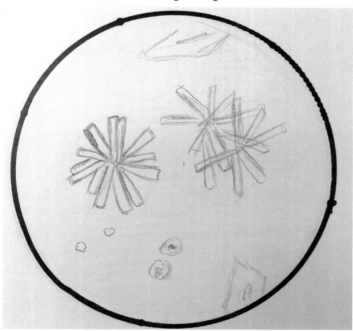

- Alkaline/neutral
- Colorless
- Solubility: dilute acetic acid

Picture 17 - Triple phosphates

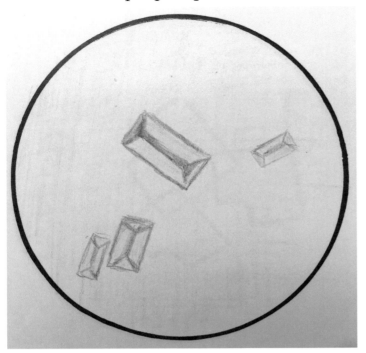

- Alkaline pH
- Colorless, coffin lids
- Solubility: dilute acetic acid

Picture 18 - Ammonium biurate

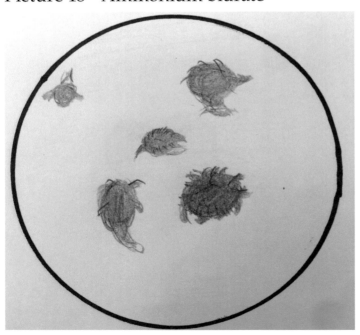

- Alkaline pH
- Yellow-brown, thorny apples
- Solubility: acetic acid with heat

Picture 19 - Calcium carbonate

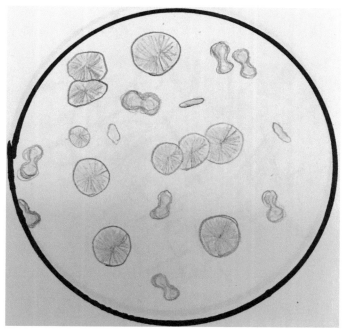

- Alkaline pH
- Colorless, dumbbells
- Solubility: gas from acetic acid

CRYSTALS (ABNORMAL)
Picture 20 - Cystine

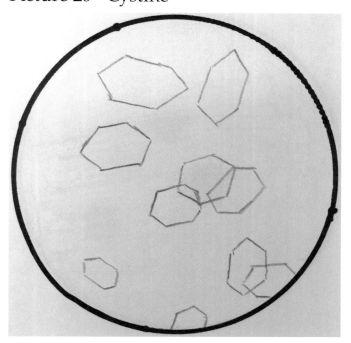

- Acid pH
- Colorless
- Solubility: ammonia, dilute HCl

Picture 21 - Cholesterol

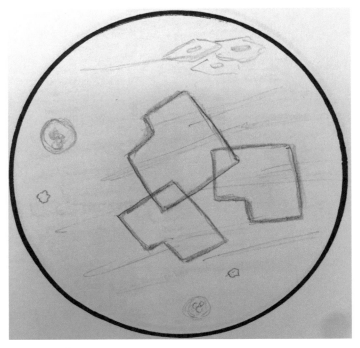

- Acid pH
- Colorless (notch plates)
- Solubility: chloroform

Picture 22 - Leucine

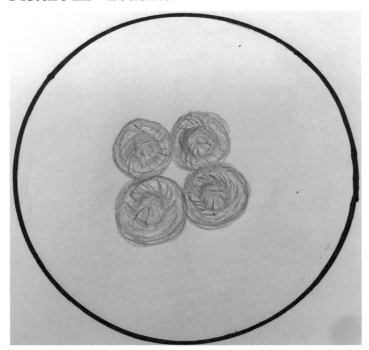

- Acid pH
- Yellow
- Solubility: hot alkali or alcohol

Picture 23 - Tyrosine

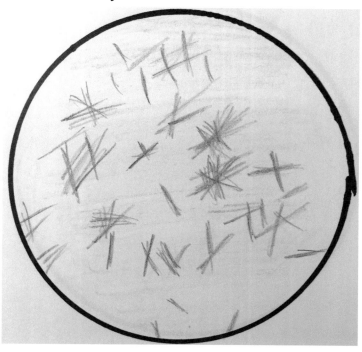

- Acid/neutral pH
- Colorless-yellow
- Solubility: alkali or heat

Picture 24 - Bilirubin

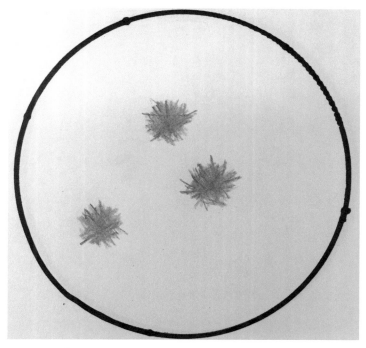

- Acid pH
- Yellow
- Solubility: acetic acid, HCl, NaOH, ether, chloroform

Picture 25 - Sulfonamides

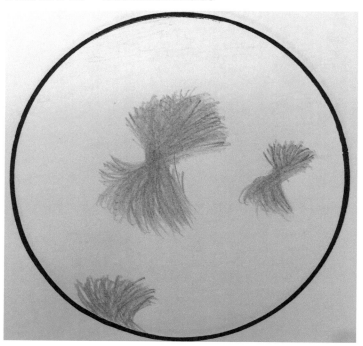

- Acid/neutral pH
- Green
- Solubility: acetone

Picture 26 - Radiographic dye

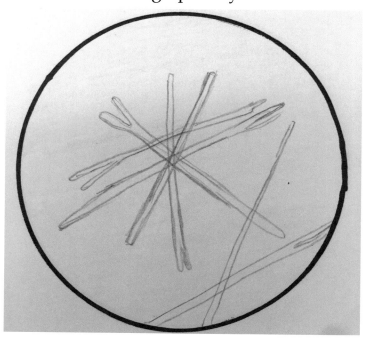

- Acid pH
- Colorless
- Solubility: 10% NaOH

Picture 27 - Ampicillin

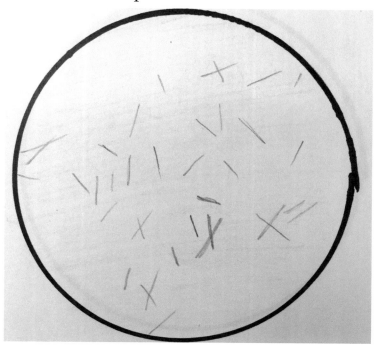

- Acid/neutral pH
- Colorless
- Refrigeration forms bundles

CELLS
Picture 28 - WBCs

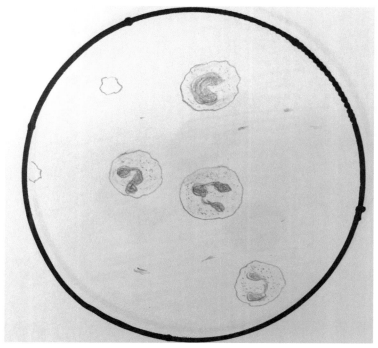

- Nucleated cells
- Reference range: ≤ 5/hpf

Picture 29 - RBCs

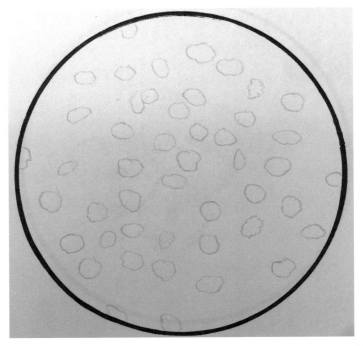

- Fragile, non-nucleated with a central pallor
- Reference range: ≤ 3/hpf

Epithelial cells
Picture 30 - Squamous epithelial cells

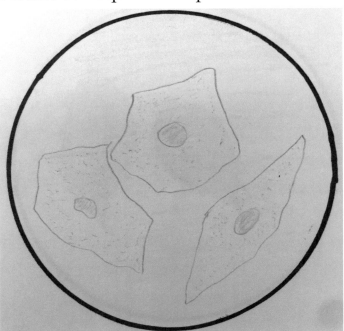

- Thin, flat, usually with angular or irregular outline and a small, round nucleus
- Reference range: normally seen in lower numbers and usually a contamination from the genital tract

Picture 31 - Transitional epithelial cells

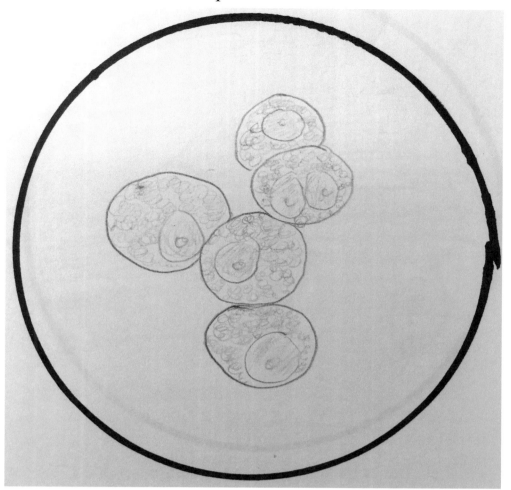

- Originates from renal pelvis ureters, bladder and/or urethra. Their size and shape depends on the depth of origin in the epithelial mucosa, most often they are round or polygonal, less commonly pear-shaped, caudate, or spindle-shaped. They are somewhat smaller and smoother than squamous cells but larger than a WBC. They may develop refractile, fatty inclusions as they degenerate in older specimens. The presence of transitional sheets "brick wall" appearance is sometimes associated with Transitional Cell Cancer (TCC)
- Reference range: <2/hpf

Picture 32 - Renal Tubular Cells (RTC)

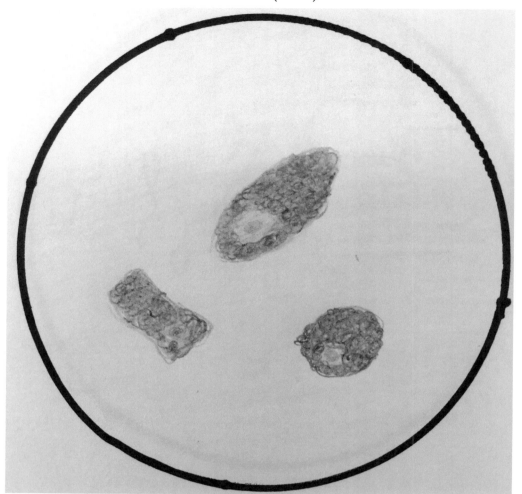

- Are originally cubic in shape but once exfoliated, they adopt a rounded shape. These cells are slightly larger than leukocytes with lightly granular cytoplasm. The nucleus is round, well defined, usually centric. The cytoplasm often shows a perinuclear halo when stained. An increase in number is seen in nephrotic syndrome and in conditions leading to a tubular degeneration. When lipiduria occurs, these cells contain endogenous fats. When filled with numerous fat droplets, such cells are called oval fat bodies. Oval fat bodies exhibit a "maltese cross" configuration by polarized light microscopy.

Picture 33 - Clue Cells

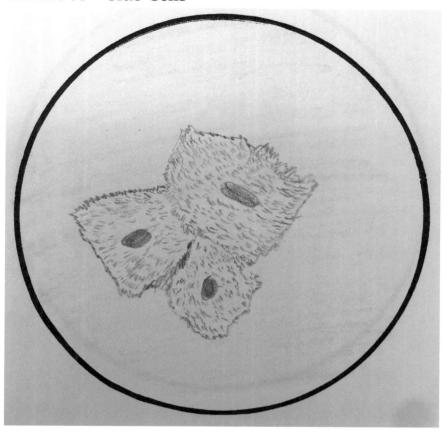

- Epithelial cells loaded with gram variable coccobacilli, Gardnerella vaginalis, an organism causing bacterial vaginosis

Picture 34 – Trichomonas (stained)

Picture 35 – Trichomonas (unstained)

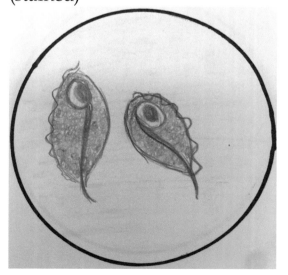
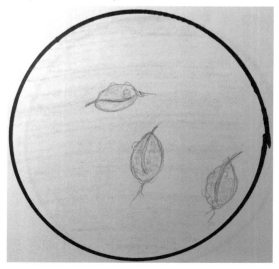

- Identification will only be performed if the organism is moving
- When the organism is dead, it resembles a large WBC

Picture 36 - Sperm

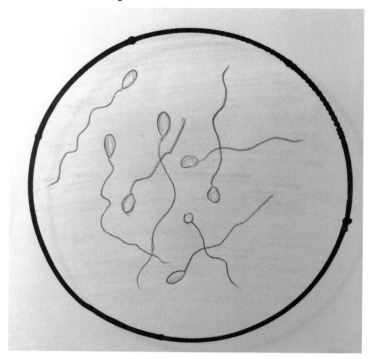

- We do not report the presence of sperm

Picture 37 – Eosinophils (10x)

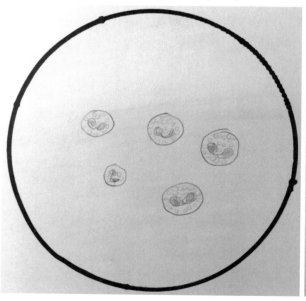

Picture 38 – Eosinophils (100x)

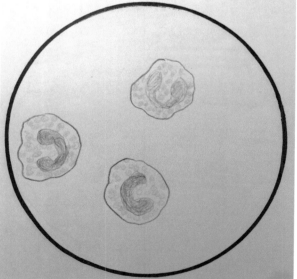

- Seen in tubulointerstitial disease associated with hypersensitivity to penicillin and its derivatives
- Allergic interstitial nephritis (along with RBCs)
- Difficult to visualize in routine microscopic examination of urine. A cytocentrifuge preparation and using a regular blood stain such as a Wright's stain can be used to examine for eosinophils

PICTURE 39 - Bacteria

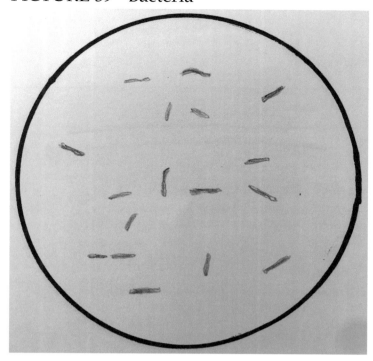

- Are reported as rare, few, moderate and many or 1+, 2+, 3+, 4+
- Reference range: rare-few (<1+)

Picture 40 - Yeast

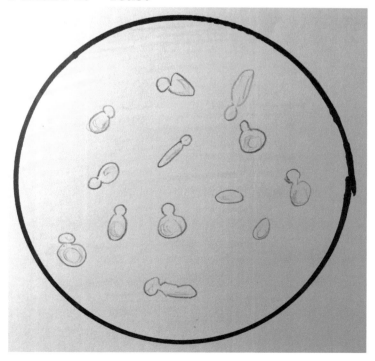

- Budding makes it easier to identify, non-budding yeasts could be mistaken for RBCs
- Seen in yeast infection

SECTION VII: Test Limitations

Table 1 Urine chemistry test limitations

Analyte	False Negative	False Positive
Glucose	Increase ascorbic acid	Presence of oxidizing substances such as chlorine or hypochlorite and pH<4.0
Protein	Urine with pH<3.0	Urine with large amount of Hgb, pH>8.0, contrast medium, disinfectants including quaternary ammonium compounds
Bilirubin	Ascorbic acid, uric acid and nitrites	Presence of urobilinogen
Urobilinogen	N/A	Presence of carbapenem
Blood	Urine with elevated specific gravity, protein or ascorbic acid	Presence of oxidizing substances such as chlorine or hypochlorite
Ketone	N/A	Drugs such as L-Dopa, phenylketone, cephalosporin, aldose, reductive anti-enzyme
Nitrite	Urine with elevated specific gravity, or ascorbic acid	N/A
Leukocytes	Urine with glucose>500, protein>300, pH 5.0 or less, elevated specific gravity	Formaldehyde
pH	N/A	N/A

SECTION VIII: Body Fluids

Urine

Aside from a routine urinalysis, urine is a body fluid that from time to time may need more extensive analysis.

1. Aminoaciduria – overflow of amino acids into the urine may be due to the following scenarios:
- Abnormal accumulation of amino acids in the blood stream that exceeds the renal threshold's capability for reabsorption due to overwhelming amount of amino acids.
- Kidney may be functioning normally but the problem is in the reabsorption.
- A breakdown in the system leads to the increase amino acids in blood and urine in the presence of normal renal clearance.
- Once substrates accumulate they may also be processed through different pathways resulting in the production of abnormal intermediates.
- The accumulated substrate and abnormal metabolites may or may not be toxic.
- Accumulation of abnormal metabolites are mainly referred to as a group of diseases called "Inborn Errors of Metabolism", where a specific enzyme deficiency results in accumulation of the substrate and the decrease or absence of the production of the product.

COMMON INBORN ERRORS OF METABOLISM
a. Phenylketonuria (PKU) – hyperphenylalaninemia, deficient in Phenylalanine Hydroxylase (PH)
  ◦ Incidence: 1:10,000-14,000 births and has 2 types
  ◦ Classic PKU (complete PH deficiency) – 1:14,000
  ◦ Variant PKU (5-20% PH deficiency) – 1:14,000
  ◦ Normal values:

Phenylalanine – (plasma: 1.2-3.4 mg/dL)	PKU patient: 15-63 mg/dL
(urine: 30mg/dL)	PKU patient: 300-1000 mg/dL
Phenylpyruvic acid – (plasma: N/A)	PKU patient: 0.3-1.8 mg/dL
(urine: N/A)	PKU patient: 300-2000 mg/dL
Phenylacetyl glutamine – urine – N/A	PKU patient: 2400 mg/dL

- ◦ Clinical significance:
  - ■ Phenylalanine accumulation in blood is toxic to developing brain. Brain damage can occur as early as the second week after birth.
  - ■ Serum phenylalaine levels of 4.5 mg/dL or higher 2-3 days after birth are considered consistent with PKU. Premies may have a slightly higher value and NOT HAVE PKU!
  - ■ Increased levels of phenylpyruvic acid and phenyl acetyl glutamine give a characteristic mousy odor to the urine.
  - ■ Untreated PKU mother can cause brain damage to a non-PKU unborn child
  - ■ PKU patients also have defect in serotonin metabolism which involves myelin synthesis. Also, melanin synthesis is affected resulting in light skin and hair
  - ■ California has a mandatory screening process for PKU of all newborns and mother with history of PKU

LABORATORY TEST: PKU
- ◦ Principle: Fluorescent
  Phenylalanine + Ninhydrin (in the presence of dipeptide L-leucine-L-alanine) → fluorescent product that is proportional to the phenylalanine concentration
  pH of 5.8
  alkaline copper tartrate – stabilizes the fluorescent product
- ◦ Principle: Colorimetric
  Ferric Chloride Test (Phenistix)
  Urine + Phosphate precipitation reagent, filter and acidify with 2-3 drops of HCl, add 2-3 drops of $FeCl_3$

  Blue-green color=positive

- ◦ Principle: Growth
  Guthrie Test
  Bacillus subtilis is placed in an agar plate with a competitive inhibitor for phenylalaine, filter paper with the patient's serum is placed onto the agar and incubated

  Bacterial growth will occur around the patient's filter paper = elevated levels of phenylalanine

b. Tyrosinuria – deficient *p*-OH-phenylpyruvic acid oxidase, resulting to elevated Tyrosine (substrate) and deficient Homogentisic acid (product)
- ◦ Clinical Significance:
  - Tyrosine, para hydroxy phenylpyruvic acid, DOPA (Dihydroxyphenylalanine), and *p*-hydroxy-phenyllactic acid accumulate in serum and spill into the urine
  - Disease results in severe liver damage and renal tubular disease
  - Incidence: Rare
  - Principle:
    Urinalysis microscopic-observance of tyrosine crystals in a feathery rosette formation

OTHER LABORATORY TESTS:
$FeCl_3$ – green color that fades rapidly
$CuSO_4$ – positive

c. Alkaptinuria
- Loss of activity of the enzyme, homogentisic acid oxidase Homogentisic acid (on the action of homogentisic acid oxidase) →Maleylacetoacetic acid
- Urine darkens upon standing
- Homogentisic acid accumulates and when exposed to air is oxidized forming a dark compound
- Patient may develop arthritis
- Incidence: Rare

d. Maple Syrup Urine Disease
- Loss of activity of oxidative decarboxylase
- Leucine, valine and isoleucine are converted to the alpha-keto acids of these amino acids by transaminases
- Lack of the oxidative decarboxylases results in the accumulation of the alpha-keto acids of these amino acids
- Principle:
  Maple Syrup Odor in the urine
  OTHER LABORATORY TESTS:
  $FeCl_3$ – green to gray color is produced
  $CuSO_4$ – negative

2. Aminoaciduria – Renal Type differs from the aminoaciduria due to the accumulation of amino acids in the blood because of the lack of specific amino acid enzymes is that the renal type have normal levels of amino acids in the blood.
- Defective tubular reabsorption resulting in increased levels of amino acids in urine
- Diseases include:
   a. Cystinuria
      - Renal transportation defect resulting in 20-30 times the normal amount of cystine in the urine. Lysine, arginine and ornithine are also excreted in increased amounts
      - May form cystine calculi
      - Except for the risk of calculi formation, this disorder is benign
      - Principle:
         Urinalysis – Cystine crystals
         OTHER LABORATORY TESTS:
         Nitroprusside test – magenta color is produced
         Lead acetate test – blackening, formation of lead sulfide (PbS)
         $FeCl_3$ – negative

   b. Hartnup Disease
      - Hereditary abnormality in the metabolism of tryptophan
      - Increased excretion of 13 amino acids
      - Faulty tubular reabsorption

LABORATORY TEST/S:
Measurement of amino acids in the urine

   c. Fanconi's Syndrome
      - Multiple hereditary abnormalities resulting in:
         - Impaired kidney function and renal hypoplasia resulting in aminoaciduria, glycinuria, cystine crystals and calculi formation
         - Pancytopenia
         - Hypogonadism
         - Mental retardation

LABORATORY TEST/S:
Measurement of amino acids, glucose, phosphate and   bicarbonate in the urine; most of these analytes are   elevated.

d. Glycinuria
- Excess urinary excretion of glycine with normal glycine concentration
- Tendency to form oxalate stones even though the quantity of urinary oxalate excretion is normal

LABORATORY TEST/S:
Glycine measurement in the urine will be elevated

3. Melanin
- Normal pigment found in hair, skin and eyes
- Patients with melanomas will produce increased amounts of a melanin precursor that darkens urine upon standing
- Principle:
  Nitroprusside – blue-black color
  $FeCl_3$ – gray-black precipitate

4. Indican
- Indole is produced by bacterial action on tryptophan in the intestine, some indole is reabsorbed into the circulation, detoxified to indican and then excreted in the urine
- Used to determine presence of bowel obstruction

LABORATORY TEST/S:
Measurement of indican in the urine.

5. 5-HIAA (5-Hydroxyindoleacetic acid)
- Serotonin is derived from tryptophan
- Serotonin metabolizes to 5-HIAA before excretion
- 5-HIAA is a smooth muscle stimulant, produced in argentaffin cells of the GI tract and transported by platelets
- Clinical Significance: carcinoid tumors
  Production of large amounts of Serotonin, resulting in large amounts of 5-HIAA

LABORATORY TEST:
Measurement of 5-HIAA in the urine

6. Oxalate
- Can be measured in serum and urine to determine an individual's likelihood to develop renal calculi

- Elevated oxalate levels are also seen after ethylene glycol (antifreeze) poisoning
- Principle:

Oxalate + O_2 (action of oxalate oxidase)$\rightarrow 2CO_2 + H_2O_2$

H_2O_2 + MBTH (action of peroxidase)$\rightarrow$Indamine dye + OH^-

*MBTH=3-methyl-2-benzothiazoline hydrazone

- Reference range: Urine 100-400 umol/L
Serum 11-27 umol/L

7. Citrate

- An inhibitor of the crystallization of calcium salts and thus helps prevent the formation of urinary calculi
- Principle:

Citrate can be measured in urine by using a series of enzymatic reactions using citrate lyase, malate dehydrogenase and lactate dehydrogenase (LDH)

The LDH reaction converts NADH to NAD which can be measured by a decrease in absorbance at 314 nm

- Reference range:
0.6-4.8 mmol/24 hrs (male)
1.3-6.0 mmol/24 hrs (female)

8. Urinary Calculi (Stones)

- The insolubility of certain compounds in the urinary tract results in the formation of kidney stones or calculi (nephrolithiasis)
- Factors that affect calculi formation include:
  - Urinary pH
  - Diet
  - Endocrine disorders (e.g. parathyroid hormone or PTH)
  - Concentrated urine (below normal urine volume)
- Principle:
  - Infrared spectrum analysis
  - X-ray diffraction
  - Chemical analysis, "stone profile" on 24-hour urine
  Oxalate
  Citrate

Uric acid
Calcium
Magnesium
Sodium
Creatinine
BUN

*Since the same preservative cannot be used for all analytes, two 24-hour collections must be obtained or a single 24-hour collection is performed and splitting the samples and adding the proper preservatives
- ➤ Dissolving and drying to determine appearance of crystals
- ➤ Visual inspection of the calculi
- ■ The following are common calculi
  - ➤ Calcium monohydrate and Calcium oxalate (acid, neutral or alkaline pH) 67.1%
  - ➤ Magnesium ammonium phosphate (alkaline pH) 19.5%
  - ➤ Uric acid (acid pH) 6.1%
  - ➤ Cystine (acid pH) 3.8%

NON-URINARY BODY FLUIDS
- • Transudate
  - a. Results from increased hydrostatic pressure
  - b. Total protein will be less than 3.0 g/dL
  - c. Seen in Congestive Heart Failure (CHF)
- • Exudate
  - a. Results from capillary permeability
  - b. Total protein will be greater than 3.0 g/dL
  - c. Seen during infections

1. Cerebrospinal Fluid (CSF)
   - • When CSF is obtained, the specimens should be used in the following order:
     Tube #1 – for chemistry (store refrigerated) and RBC count
     Tube #2 – culture (store R.T.)
     Tube #3 – cells counts and differential (store R.T.)
     *note: if 4 tubes are submitted, always use tube #2 for culture and the last tube for cell counts and differential
   - • Normal values:

Appearance	Clear
Glucose	40-80 mg/dL
Protein	12-60 mg/dL
WBCs	<5 cells/uL
RBCs	<5 cells/uL

- Appearance
  - ➤ Clear – normal
  - ➤ Hazy, turbid, cloudy, milky – WBCs and/or RBCs present, (hemorrhage, traumatic tap), microorganisms (meningitis), protein (production of IgG within central nervous system or CNS) and other disorders that affect the blood-brain barrier
  - ➤ Oily – radiographic contrast media
  - ➤ Bloody – RBCs (hemorrhage)
  - ➤ Xanthochromic (yellowish tinge) – hemoglobin (old hemorrhage, lysed cells from traumatic tap), bilirubin (RBC breakdown), merthiolate (contamination), carotene (increased serum levels), protein (IgG), melanin (meningeal melanosarcoma)
  - ➤ Clotted – protein (IgG), clotting factors (introduced by traumatic tap)
  - ➤ Pellicle (scum on the surface of the CSF) – protein (disorders that affect the blood-brain barrier), clotting factors (tubercular meningitis)
- Protein
  - ➤ Increase in tumors, infections, inflammation, injury to the spine
  - ➤ Decrease in chronic CSF leakage and water intoxication
- Glucose
  - ➤ Decrease glucose may indicate infection
  - ➤ Increase indicates diabetes

Fluid counts are performed in a Neubauer Hemocytometer (Picture 41)

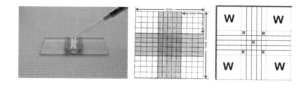

Differential counts employ the use of a cytospin and stain like a normal blood smear (Wright's stain)

Neubauer hemocytometer counting chamber is composed of 9 large squares:
1 large square = 1.0 mm
Total square volume = 0.9 ul
4 large corner squares = 0.4 ul
2 diagonal corner squares = 0.2 ul
4 corner squares of the large center square = 0.044 ul

Cell count = $\dfrac{\text{# cells counted x dilution}}{\text{Volume counted}}$

2. Synovial Fluid
- Originates from the joint
- Cells seen in synovial fluids:

  ➢ Neutrophil (polymorphonuclear leukocytes) – presence may indicate bacterial infection or crystal-induced inflammation
  ➢ Lymphocyte (mononuclear leukocyte) – presence may indicate viral infection
  ➢ Macrophage/monocyte (large mononuclear leukocyte, may be vacuolated) – elevated amount may indicate viral infection

- Crystals seen in synovial fluids:

  ➢ Monosodium urates – needle-shaped, may be intra or extracellular
  ➢ Calcium pyrophosphate – rods/needle/rhombics, intra or extracellular
  ➢ Cholesterol – notched rhombic plates, extracellular
  ➢ Uric acid – needle-shaped, may be intra or extracellular

3. Pleural fluid
- Obtained by thoracentesis from the pleural cavity (lung cavity)
- Should be examined for RBCs and WBCs
- Can also be submitted for cytology work-up to look for malignant cells

4. Semen analysis
- Should be tested for motility within 30 minutes to 1 hour of collection of the sperm or will start dying and motility test will not be accurate

- Evaluate sperm motility by placing 1 drop of semen on the slide and noting the percentage that are moving in progressive motion
- Count cellular elements by making a 1:20 dilution and counting in a Neubauer Hemocytometer
- Normal values:

Volume	2-5 ml
Viscosity	pours in droplets (not sticky)
pH	7.3-8.3
Count	20-160 mil/mL
Motility	>50-60% within 1 hour
Morphology	<30% abnormal forms

- Semen analysis may be ordered to evaluate a successful vasectomy, which is no sperm observed.

5. Amniotic fluid
- Functions as the pressure barrier for fetus and assures fetal mobility and as a waste disposal
- Composition
  - Early stages – electrolyte values much like the plasma
  - Becomes slightly hypotonic (less solute)
  - Increase in urea, creatinine and uric acid due to fetal urine
  - Protein and albumin decreases to a $1/20^{th}$ level of plasma

    - Amniocentesis
      - Slight risk of fetal injury, TREAT AMNIOTIC FLUID WITH CARE! Sample is collected by needle aspiration with the help of ultrasound
      - Physician should avoid fetal injury or contamination with maternal urine
    - Amniotic fluid – should be protected from light (will destroy bilirubin present)
    - Bilirubin and oxyhemoglobin in utero
    - Can be measured spectrophotometrically
    - Bilirubin has an absorbance peak of 450 nm
    - -Interpretation depends on weeks of gestation therefore accurate determination of weeks of gestation is important

- -increased amniotic bilirubin will occur in mothers with increased bilirubin
- -in Hemolytic Disease of the Newborn (HDN), amniotic bilirubin is requested if maternal anti-D titer is >1:16
- Oxyhemoglobin has an absorption peak of 410 nm
- -intact RBCs in amniotic fluid must be identified as the mother or the fetus by Anti-Globulin Test (AGT), Rh (if Rh incompatibility is established) or Kleihauer-Betke Test or Test for Fetal Hemoglobin
- -if the blood is identified as that of fetal, then there is fetal bleeding
- Meconium Staining (fetal intestinal discharge)
  - ➤ Meconium is a thick green tar-like substance that lines the baby's intestines during pregnancy. Typically this is not release in the baby's bowel movement until after birth. Occasionally a baby will have a bowel movement prior to birth excreting the meconium in the amniotic fluid
  - ➤ if present in amniotic fluid, especially in later gestation, indicates fetal stress
  - ➤ May mask HDN because of the presence of bilirubin in meconium
  - ➤ Meconium gives a green color to amniotic fluid and gives it an opaque appearance

- Creatinine
  - ➤ Useful in ruling out maternal urine (contamination in the collection of amniotic fluid)
- L/S ratio – Lecithin to Sphingomyelin Ratio
  - ➤ Lecithin is a surfactant and is needed in the newborn lung so that the lungs will be able to exchange CO_2 with oxygen in the air
  - ➤ The ratio of lecithin to sphingomyelin is a good indicator of fetal lung maturity
  - ➤ If the L/S ratio is >2:1 then the lung is considered mature enough
  - ➤ If the L/S ratio is <1:1 then there is a risk of the fetus getting hyaline membrane disease (respiratory distress syndrome)
  - ➤ The ratio is useful when the physician is considering inducing the patient for early delivery due to other causes or to hold off delivery to allow the lung to mature

- ➢ Principle:
- ➢ Thin Layer Chromatography (TLC) – false maturity ratio may occur with diabetic mothers
- ◦ Phosphatidyl Glycerol (PG)
  - ➢ Not present until lungs have matured and therefore more specific than L/S ratio
  - ➢ Performed by TLC or other immunoassay procedure
  - ➢ Disaturated Phosphatidylcholine (DSPC)
  - ➢ 85% of total lecithin in fetal lungs
  - ➢ Measured semi-quantitatively by reacting phospholipid extract of amniotic fluid with Osmium tetroxide
- ◦ Micro-viscosity by Fluorescence Polarization
  - ➢ Phospholipids are tagged with fluorescent marker. Surfactants from the amniotic fluid from fetus with mature lungs will lower the micro-viscosity and increase the rotation of the marker
  - ➢ Bed-side shake test
  - ➢ Bubble stability is related to surfactant present. This test is used only in an emergency basis when TLC is not available.
  - ➢ Amniotic fluid is mixed with 95% ethanol, appearance of bubbles indicates presence of surfactants and the lungs can survive outside of the womb. This test is also called Bubble Stability Test or Rapid Surfactant Test

*Note: Hemolysis will cause variable results

URINALYSIS - WRITTEN EXAMINATION

(25 Points)

(Please circle the correct answer)

1. A crystal that is expected to be found in lipoid nephrosis is:

a.

b.

c.

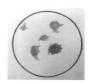
d.

2. Large amounts of Vitamin C ingested by a patient who submits a urine specimen for urinalysis will affect the dipstick test in the following manner:
   a. Glucose oxidase method causing a falsely lowered value
   b. Glucose oxidase method causing a falsely elevated value
   c. Occult blood causing a falsely elevated value
   d. Reducing sugars (Benedict's test) causing a falsely decrease value

3. The reagent most commonly used in testing for ketone bodies is most sensitive to the presence of the following substance:
   a. Acetone
   b. Acetoacetic acid
   χ. γ-Hydroxybutyric acid
   d. hemoglobin

4. A test for occult blood on urine was performed and a positive result was obtained on the dipstick test. Microscopic examination revealed no red blood cells. Addition of ammonium sulfate was negative for precipitation. The substance giving the positive result is most likely:
   a. Hemoglobin
   b. Myoglobin
   c. Cast
   d. Mucoprotein

5. A young adult male complains of dysuria with burning. Urinalysis results are:

   Nitrite: Positive
   Protein: Positive

   pH: 8.5

   Others within normal range

   Many WBCs/hpf

   Gram stain: Gram negative intracellular diplococci

   The patient probably has:

   a. Acute glomerulonephritis
   b. Streptococcal cystitis
   c. Gonorrheal urethritis
   d. Syphilis

6. A patient presents with fever, bilateral flank pain and mild to moderate proteinuria and urine sediment that contains leukocyte casts and granular casts, occasional RBCs, many bacteria and neutrophil. The findings point toward:
   a. Acute pyelonephritis
   b. Acute glomerulonephritis
   c. Bladder cancer
   d. Nephrotic syndrome

7. pH is most commonly measured by the urine dipstick method using which of the following reagents:
   a. Ehrlich's reagent
   b. P-nitrobenzene diazonium-p-toluene sulfonate

    c. Bromthymol blue

    d. Diacetyl reagent

8. The normal range for specific gravity on a random urine sample is:

    a. 0.900-0.950

    b. 1.000-1.050

    c. 1.003-1.030

    d. 1.100-1.200

9. A patient has symptoms of a urinary tract infection and a first morning random urine was submitted to the laboratory. Dipstick tests demonstrate:

    A pH = 8.0

    Protein = positive

    Blood = negative

    Nitrite = negative

    Leukocyte = positive

    Microscopic analysis reveals many bacteria and WBCs

Based on these results, the UTI may be caused by:

    a. Staphylococcus saprophyticus

    b. E. coli

    c. Klebsiella pneumonia

    d. Proteus vulgaris

10. A negative glucose oxidase test and a positive Benedict's test WOULD NOT BE caused by which of the following:

    a. Galactose

    b. Lactose

    c. Fructose

    d. Glucose

11. A positive dipstick protein was negative in sulfosalicylic acid, what could be the most likely cause of the dipstick positive?

    a. Ascorbic acid

    b. pH >8.0

    c. pH<6.0

    d. bacteria

12. An elevated number of this cell may indicate Transitional Cell Carcinoma:

    a. Clue cells

    b. Epithelial cells

    c. Renal tubular epithelial cells

    d. Transitional epithelial cells

13. The following crystals are normally found in a non-fresh urine except:
   a. Uric acid crystals
   b. Triple phosphate crystals
   c. Tyrosine crystals
   d. Calcium oxalate crystals

14. The presence of this cast may indicate glomerulonephritis:

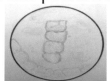
a.

b.

c.

d.

15. The Benedict's test contains copper sulfate, sodium hydroxide and sodium carbonate with a specific test for this carbohydrate:
   a. Glucose
   b. Lactose
   c. Sucrose
   d. Galactose

16. Bence-Jones protein precipitates between what temperature?
   a. 20-40°C
   b. 30-50°C
   c. 40-60°C
   d. 60-80°C

17. A 1-week old baby tested positive on the glucose dipstick, what test should confirm this?
   a. Sulfosalycilic acid
   b. Ketostix

    c. Clinitest

    d. Ictotest

18. The amount of protein suggestive of renal proteinuria is:

    a. <1g/day

    b. 1-4 g/day

    c. >4g/day

    d. >10g/day

19. This disaccharide is made up of glucose and galactose:

    a. Maltose

    b. Lactose

    c. Fructose

    d. Sucrose

20. A positive bilirubin test should be confirmed with:

    a. Ictotest

    b. Ketostix

    c. Clinitest

    d. TCA

21. A bacterially metabolized direct bilirubin that is soluble in chloroform:

    a. Porphobilinogen

    b. Coproporphrinogen

    c. Protoporphrinogen

    d. Urobilinogen

22. When the body depletes glucose, the body start breaking down fats and these starts appearing in the urine:

    a. Proteins

    b. Ketones

    c. Calcium

    d. Phosphates

23. The following crystal is found in the acid urine:

    a. Calcium phosphatase

    b. Triple phosphates

    c. Amorphous urates

    d. Calcium carbonates

24. The following cannot be detected in the dipstick except in microscopic exam:
    a. WBC
    b. RBC
    c. Yeast
    d. Bacteria
25. Aside from Specific Gravity, this also measures the total quantity of solutes in the urine:
    a. pH
    b. Osmolality
    c. Cardiolipin
    d. Phospholipid

Urinalysis Written Exam Answer Key

1. b
2. a
3. b
4. a
5. c
6. a
7. c
8. c
9. a
10. d
11. b
12. d
13. c
14. b
15. d
16. c
17. c
18. a
19. b
20. a
21. d
22. b
23. c
24. c
25. b

BODY FLUIDS - WRITTEN EXAMINATION

(20 Points)

(Please circle the correct answer)

1. Which of the following lecithin/sphingomyelin (L/S) ratios performed on amniotic fluid would indicate fetal lung maturity in a non-hemolyzed, non-diabetic patient:
   a. 0.5:1
   b. 1:1
   c. 1.5:1
   d. 3.5:1
2. In case of bacterial meningitis, the cerebrospinal fluid glucose is _____, and the cerebrospinal fluid protein is _____.
   a. Increased, increased
   b. Increased, decreased
   c. Decreased, increased
   d. Decreased, decreased
3. The following results were obtained from the analysis of a fresh CSF specimen:

Protein:	80 mg/dL
Serum glucose:	103 mg/dL
CSF glucose:	20 mg/dL
WBC:	1200 cells/ul (90% neutrophils)
RBC:	600 cells/uL
India Ink Stain:	Negative

   This indicates the following type of infection:
   a. Bacterial
   b. Cryptococcus infection
   c. Viral infection
   d. No infection, specimen contaminated with blood
4. Phenylketonuria is caused by a deficiency of the enzyme:
   a. Phenylpyruvic acid oxidase
   b. Phenylalanine hydroxylase
   c. Phenylacetic glutamine deaminase
   d. Homogentisic acid oxidase

5. This analyte is not present until the lungs have matured and therefore more specific than L/S ratio:
   a. Disaturated Phosphatidylcholine (DSPC)
   b. Phosphatidyl Glycerol (PG)
   c. Oxyhemoglobin
   d. Bilirubin
6. In normal individual, the CSF glucose concentration is approximately _____ that of the blood glucose level
   a. 25%
   b. 33%
   c. 66%
   d. 90%
7. The hereditary abnormality in the metabolism of tryptophan which increases the excretion of 13 amino acids is a characteristic of this disease:
   a. Hartnup disease
   b. Maple syrup disease
   c. Glycinuria
   d. Fanconi's syndrome
8. A fresh CSF specimen was brought to the laboratory. After centrifugation, the supernatant was clear and yellow. The spinal fluid:
   a. Is normal, CSF is normally yellow
   b. Was not drawn carefully, blood contaminated the specimen during collection
   c. Possible old hemorrhage in the CSF has occurred
   d. Shows that bacterial infection of the meninges has taken place
9. The elevated serotonin could be measured by measuring:
   a. Indican
   b. Tryptophan
   c. 5-HIAA
   d. Citrate
10. What disorder would cause a darkening of the urine upon standing?
   a. Phenylketonuria
   b. Alkaptinuria
   c. Cystinuria
   d. Tyrosinuria
   e. Glycinuria
11. These analytes give a characteristic mousy odor to the urine:
   a. Phenylpyruvic acid
   b. Phenylacetylglutamine

c. Phenylpyruvic oxidase
d. Phenhydrazone
e. a and b
f. a and c
g. a and d
h. b and c
i. b and d
j. c and d

12. This test determines the presence of bowel obstruction by measuring the increase in:
    a. Indican
    b. 5-HIAA
    c. Tryptophan
    d. Melanin

13. Elevated melanin will produce what color with the nitroprusside test:
    a. Blue-black
    b. Blue-green
    c. Reddish-black
    d. Blue-gray

14. The sweet smell in the urine in the Maple syrup disease is caused by the accumulation of:
    a. Phenylpyruvic acid
    b. Phenylalanine
    c. Homogentisic
    d. Alpha keto acids

15. The defficiency in p-OH-phenylpyruvic acid oxidase causes the disorder:
    a. Phenylketonuria
    b. Alkaptinuria
    c. Tyrosinuria
    d. Cystinuria

16. An elevated oxalate determines:
    a. A likelihood in developing crystals
    b. A likelihood in developing casts
    c. A likelihood in developing amino acids
    d. A likelihood in developing renal stones

17. Factors that affect calculi formation include all except:
    a. Endocrine disorders
    b. Diet
    c. Production of 5-HIAA
    d. pH
18. The least isolated renal stone is:
    a. Cystine
    b. Uric acid
    c. Calcium monohydrate
    d. Magnesium ammonium phosphate
19. A synovial fluid was collected from a patient suffering from extreme joint pain, the RA and culture was negative. The notched rhombic plate structure observed extracellularly in the fluid is most probably that of:
    a. Monosodium urates
    b. Cholesterol
    c. Uric acid
    d. Calcium pyrophosphates
20. Semen analysis should be perform within 30 minutes to 1 hour of collection because:
    a. It will falsely elevate the count
    b. It will falsely decrease the count
    c. It will falsely decrease motility
    d. It will falsely increase abnormal morphology

Body Fluid Written Exam Answer Key

1. d
2. c
3. a
4. b
5. b
6. c
7. a
8. c
9. c
10. b
11. e
12. a
13. a
14. d
15. c
16. d
17. c
18. a
19. b
20. c

Afterword

In a perfect world, after their clinical rotation, CLSs and MLTs will be working in all four areas of study of medical technology or clinical science (Microbiology, Chemistry, Hematology and Immunohematology), retain all that they know and live and work happily ever after. But as we all know that is far from the case, more frequently than not, a CLS or MLT will be stuck in one or two specialized area of study. Urinalysis and body fluids is a unique sub-specialty of the department of Hematology. Urinalysis is one of the most common test offered in practically every hospital while examination of body fluids, and in particular, cerebrospinal fluid or CSF have to be done immediately because physicians have to rule out acute meningitis.

CLSs who had been away from the hematology/urinalysis/body fluids department for a period of time or never had the chance to work in this department will need a good refresher course before venturing into this department. This manual does not claim to boost someone's confidence overnight or claim to have all the answers, but instead this manual serves as a guide to re-discovering what one previously knew.

In addition to serving as a refresher course, this manual can also serve as a reviewer for CLS and MLT students at or nearing their clinical rotation as well as those taking the CLS and MLT State or National licenses.

My hope is that this manual will serve its purpose and be a source of confidence to those who are contemplating to work in the hematology/urinalysis/body fluids department as a newbee or someone who had been away from it for a period of time.

Glossary

ACUTE PORPHYRIA – an autosomal dominant porphyria that is due to a deficiency of hydroxymethylbilane synthase in the liver, the third enzyme in the 8-enzyme biosynthetic pathway of heme.

ALDOSE – an enzyme of the lyase class that catalyzes the cleavage of fructose 1,6-biphosphatase to form dihydroxyacetone phosphate and glyceraldehyde 3-phosphate.

ALKALOSIS – a pathological condition that removes acid or adds base to the body fluids.

AMINO ACIDS – organic compounds that generally contain an amino ($-NH_2$) and a carboxyl (-COOH) group.

AMNIOCENTESIS – percutaneous transabdominal puncture of the uterus during pregnancy to obtain amniotic fluid. It is commonly used for fetal karotype determination in order to diagnose abnormal fetal conditions.

ANTIDEURETIC HORMONES – released by the neurohypophysis of all vertebrates (structure varies with species) to regulate water balance and osmolarity.

ASCORBIC ACID – a 6-carbon compound related to glucose found naturally in citrus fruits and many vegetables.

BILIVERDIN – 1,3,6,7-tetramethyl-4,5-dicarboxyethyl-2,8-divinylbilenone. Biosynthesized from hemoglobin as a precursor of bilirubin.

CITRATE LYASE – an enzyme that, in the presence of ATP and Coenzyme A, catalyzes the cleavage of citrate to yield Acetyl CoA, Oxaloacetate, ADP, and orthophosphate.

DIAZONIUM – the monovalent cation N_2^+ that is composed of 2 nitrogen atoms united to carbon in an organic radical that usually exists in salts used in the manufacture of azo dyes.

EXUDATES – are fluids, cells, or other cellular substances that are slowly discharged from blood vessels usually from inflamed tissues.

GLUCOSE-6-PHOSPHATE DEHYDROGENASE DEFICIENCY – an enzyme found in red blood cells that dehydrogenates glucose-6-phosphate in a glucose degradation pathway alternative to the Kreb's cycle.

GLUCOSURIA – the presence in the urine of abnormal amounts of sugar.

GLYCINURIA – a kidney disorder characterized by the presence of excessive amounts of glycine in the urine.

GOODPASTEUR'S SYNDROME – an autoimmune disorder of unknown cause characterized by the presence of circulating antibodies in the blood which attack the basement membrane of the kidney's glomeruli and the lung's alveoli and that is marked initially by coughing, fatigue, difficulty in breathing, and hemoptysis progressing to glomerulonephritis and pulmonary hemorrhages.

HEMOCHROMATOSIS – a hereditary disorder of metabolism involving the deposition of iron-containing pigments in the tissues that is characterized especially by joint or abdominal pain, weakness, and fatigue and that may lead to bronzing of the skin, arthritis, diabetes, cirrhosis, or heart disease if untreated.

HEREDITARY SPHEROCYTOSIS – a disorder of red blood cells that is inherited as a dominant trait and is characterized by anemia, small thick fragile spherocytes which are extremely susceptible to hemolysis, enlargement of the spleen, reticulocytosis, and mild jaundice.

HOMOGENTISIC ACID - a chrystalline acid $C_8H_8O_4$ formed as an intermediate in the metabolism of phenylalanine and tyrosine and found especially in the urine of those affected with alkaptonuria.

HYPOKALEMIA – a deficiency of potassium in the blood.

HYPOGONADISM – condition resulting from deficient gonadal functions, such as gametogenesis and the production of gonadal steroid hormones. It is characterized by delay in growth, germ cell maturation, and development of secondary sex characteristics.

HYPOPLASIA – a condition of arrested development in which an organ or part remains below the normal size or an immature state.

INDICAN – a substance occurring in the urines of mammals and also in blood plasma as the normal metabolite of tryptophan.

L-DIHYDROXYPHENYLALANINE – L-3,4 dihydroxyphenylalanine is the naturally occurring form of dihydroxyphenylalanine and the immediate precursor of dopamine.

LACTATE DEHYDROGENASE – a tetrameric enzyme that, along with the coenzyme NAD+, catalyzes the interconversion of lactate and pyruvate.

MALATE DEHYDROGENASE – an enzyme that catalyzes the conversion of (S)-malate and NAD+ to oxaloacetate and NADH.

4-MALEYLACETOACETIC ACID – is an intermediate in the metabolism of tyrosine.

MARCH HEMOGLOBINURIA – hemolysis caused by repeated uncushioned shocks or trauma to some body part, such as in some soldiers on long marches, in marathon runners, and in karate practitioners.

MELANIN – insoluble polymers of tyrosine derivatives found in and causing darkness in skin (skin pigmentation), hair, and feathers providing protection against sunburn induced by sunlight.

MELANOSARCOMA – a benign or malignant skin tumor containing dark pigment.

METABOLIC SYNDROME – a syndrome marked by the presence of usually three or more of a group of factors (such as high blood pressure, abdominal obesity, high triglyceride levels, low HDL levels, and high fasting levels of blood sugar) that are linked to increased risk of cardiovascular disease and type 2 diabetes – called also insulin resistance syndrome.

METABOLITE – a product of metabolism.

METHEMOGLOBIN – a soluble brown christalline basic blood pigment that differs from hemoglobin in containing ferric iron and in being unable to combine reversibly with molecular oxygen.

MULTIPLE MYELOMA – a disease of bone marrow that is characterized by the presence of numerous myelomas in various bones of the body.

MYOGLOBIN – a red iron-containing protein pigment in muscles that is similar to hemoglobin.

NEPHROLITHIASIS – a condition marked by the presence of renal calculi.

NEPHROTIC SYNDROME – an abnormal condition that is marked by deficiency of albumin in the blood and its excretion in the urine due to altered permeability of the glomerular basement membranes.

NITROPRUSSIDE TEST – also known as sodium cyanide nitroprusside test is a rapid, simple, and qualitative determination of cystine concentrations.

OXYHEMOGLOBIN – hemoglobin loosely combined with oxygen that it releases to the tissues.

PANCYTOPENIA – an abnormal reduction of erythrocytes, white blood cells, and blood platelets in the blood.

PAROXYSMAL COLD HEMOGLOBINURIA – a condition characterized by the recurrence of hemoglobinuria caused by intravascular hemolysis occurring upon cold exposure.

PERINUCLEAR – situated around or surrounding the nucleus of a cells.

PERITUBULAR – being adjacent to or around a tubule.

PINOCYTOSIS – the uptake of fluid and dissolved substances by a cell by invagination and pinching off of the cell membrane.

PHENOLPHTHALEIN – a white or yellowish-white chrystalline compound $C_{20}H_{14}O_4$ used in analysis as an indicator because its solution is brilliant red in alkalines and is decolorized by acids and in medicine as a laxative.

PHENYLKETONURIA – an inherited metabolic disorder by an enzyme deficiency resulting in accumulation of phenylalanine and its metabolites in the blood causing usually severe mental retardation and seizures unless phenylalanine is restricted from the diet beginning at birth.

PHENYLPYRUVIC ACID – a chrystalline keto acid $C_9H_8O_3$ found in the urine as a metabolic product of phenylalanine especially in phenylketonuria.

POLYELECTROLYTE – a substance of high molecular weight (such as a protein) that is an electrolyte.

PORPHOBILINOGEN – a dicarboxylic acid C10H14N2O4 that is derived from pyrrole, that is found in the urine in acute porphyria, and that on condensation of four molecules yields uroporphyrin and other porphyrins.

PORPHYRIN – any of various compounds with a macrocyclic structure that consists essentially of four pyrrole rings joined by four =CH- groups; especially: one (such as chlorophyll or hemoglobin) containing a central metal atom and usually exhibiting biological activity.

PROSTATITIS – inflammation of the prostate glands.

PYELOGRAPHY – radiographic visualization of the renal pelvis of a kidney after injection of a radiopaque substance through the ureter or into a vein.

QUATERNARY AMMONIUM COMPOUNDS – derivative of ammonium compounds, NH_4+ Y-, in which all 4 of the hydrogens bonded to nitrogen replaced with hydrocarbyl groups.

RHOMBIC – having the form of rhombus, a parallelogram with 4 equal sides and sometimes one with no right angles.

SCHISTOSOMIASIS – infestation caused by schistosomes; specifically: a severe endemic disease of humans in Africa and parts of Asia and South America that is contracted when cercariae released into fresh waters (such as rivers) by a snail intermediate host penetrate the skin and that is marked especially by blood loss and tissue damage – called also snail fever.

SOLUTE – a dissolved substance.

TOLBUTAMIDE – a sulfonylurea $C_{12}H_{18}N_2O_3$ used in the treatment of diabetes.

TRANSUDATES – are fluids that pass through a membrane or squeeze through tissue or into the extracellular space of tissues. Transudates are thin and watery and contain few cells or proteins.

TRYPTOPHAN – an essential amino acid that is necessary for normal growth in infants and for nitrogen balance in adults. It is a precursor of serotonin (hence its use as an antidepressant and sleep aid).

TUBULOINTERSTITIAL DISEASE – disease affecting or involving the tubules and interstitial tissue of the kidney.

URETHRITIS – inflammation of the urethra.

UROBILINOGEN – a colorless compound formed in the intestines by the reduction of bilirubin.

VASECTOMY – surgical removal of the ductus deferens, or a portion of it.

REFERENCES:

1. Strassinger, S.K. and Di Lorenzo, M.S. (2014). Urinalysis and Body Fluids, 6th Edition. Philadelphia, PA. F.A. Davis Company.
2. Kaplan, A., Jack, R., Opheim, K.E., Toivola, B. and Lyon, A.W. (1995). Clinical Chemistry Interpretation and Techniques, 4th Edition. Malvern, PA. Williams and Wilkins.
3. Tietz, N. Ed. (1976). Fundamentals of Clinical Chemistry. Philadelphia, PA. W.B. Saunders Company.
4. https://www.merriam-webster.com/
5. www.online-medical-dictionary.org/

About the Author

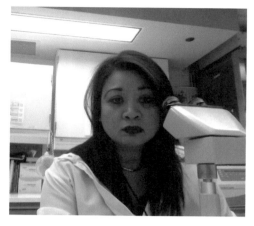

Mary Michelle Shodja earned her Bachelors of Science Degree in Medical Technology in 1992 from California State University (CSU) Dominguez Hills in Carson, California. She took her medical technology clinical year training from the Southern California Kaiser Permanente Medical Hospital and Regional Laboratory. She earned her Masters of Science Degree in Bioanalysis in 1995 from her alma mater CSU Dominguez Hills and her PhD in Epidemiology from Loma Linda University School of Public Health in 2017.

She gained Certifications in both the MLS American Society of Clinical Pathologists (ASCP) and CLS National Credentialing Agency (NCA) in 1993. Her professional career includes working in the Microbiology department at the Southern California Kaiser Permanente Regional Laboratory and as a generalist in various hospitals working in Hematology, Chemistry, Serology, Immunology and Blood Bank. She also worked for 4 years as a Microbiology laboratory instructor at Loma Linda University School of Allied Health.

Over the years she took on managerial, supervisory, teaching and other administrative and consultative work but her real passion lies in the clinical bench work and teaching. Earning her PhD in Epidemiology she plans to integrate her clinical laboratory knowledge to helping lower disease burdens globally.

Printed in the United States
By Bookmasters